The Purpose of this Book

Every year thousands of people including doctors, medical students, paramedics, nurses, nursing students, and others involved in the care and treatment of cardiac patients, get introduced to the world of reading electrocardiograms (ECGs or EKGs).

This skill is fundamental to understanding if a patient is having a problem with the rhythm of their heart, has an electrolyte problem, is receiving too much of a given medication, experiencing an infection or inflammation of the heart, has too much fluid around the heart, or are experiencing a myocardial infarction.

While reading an electrocardiogram may seem daunting at first, this book was designed from my lectures used to train students, interns, residents and fellows, on how to read an electrocardiogram. Rather than memorizing facts, this book will walk you through the steps of how to read electrocardiograms from beginning to end using the same approach used by Cardiologists like myself.

In Part 3 of How to Read an Electrocardiogram, we will look at a series of three lectures given by myself to my medical students, residents and fellows; on the Basics of ECG rhythms and axis orientation, Basic Rhythm interpretation and problems, and finally Dysrhythmias.

If you learn nothing else, please learn we are not talking about arrhythmias. "A" means the absence of something so the only "arrhythmia" is "asystole" or the absence of a rhythm. Everything else is a "dys" or "abnormal" rhythm; aka "dysrhythmia."

How to Read Electrocardiograms -

Part 3: Basic ECGs, Basic Rhythm Problems & Dysrhythmias.

By: Dr. Richard M. Fleming

Physicist – Nuclear Cardiologist

EKG Basics

By: Dr. Richard M. Fleming

Physicist – Nuclear Cardiologist

Outline

1. Review of the conduction system
2. EKG waveforms and intervals
3. EKG leads
4. Determining heart rate
5. Determining QRS axis

The Normal Conduction System

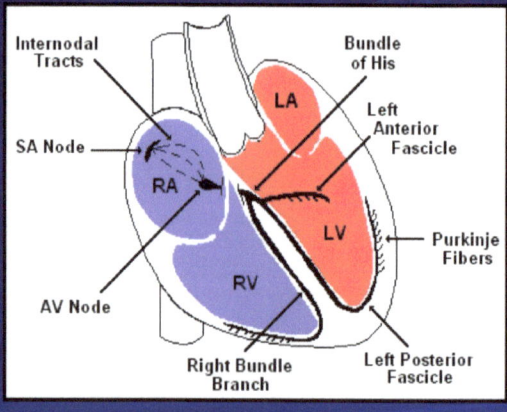

What is an EKG?

The electrocardiogram (EKG) is a representation of the electrical events of the cardiac cycle.

Each event has a distinctive waveform, the study of which can lead to greater insight into a patient's cardiac pathophysiology.

What types of pathology can we identify and study from EKGs?

- Arrhythmias
- Myocardial ischemia and infarction
- Pericarditis
- Chamber hypertrophy
- Electrolyte disturbances (i.e. hyperkalemia, hypokalemia)
- Drug toxicity (i.e. digoxin and drugs which prolong the QT interval)

Waveforms and Intervals

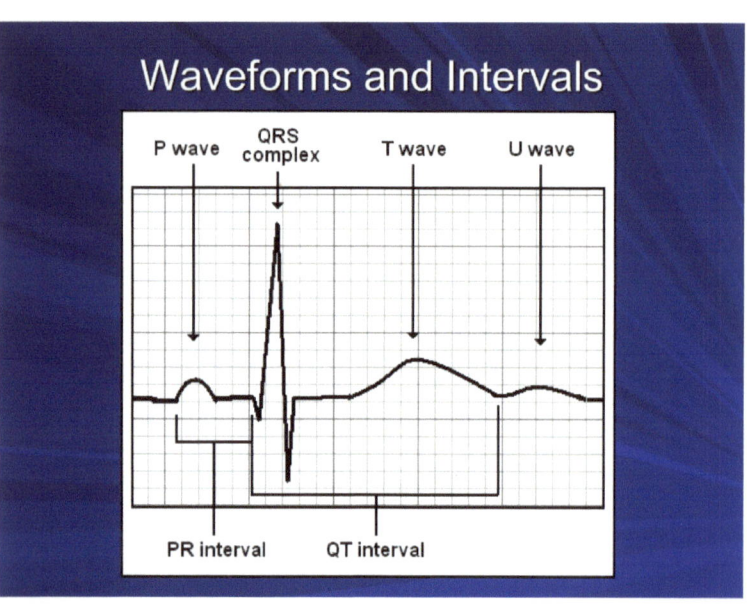

EKG Leads

Leads are electrodes which measure the difference in electrical potential between either:

1. Two different points on the body (bipolar leads)

2. One point on the body and a virtual reference point with zero electrical potential, located in the center of the heart (unipolar leads)

EKG Leads

The standard EKG has 12 leads:
- 3 Standard Limb Leads
- 3 Augmented Limb Leads
- 6 Precordial Leads

The axis of a particular lead represents the viewpoint from which it looks at the heart.

Standard Limb Leads

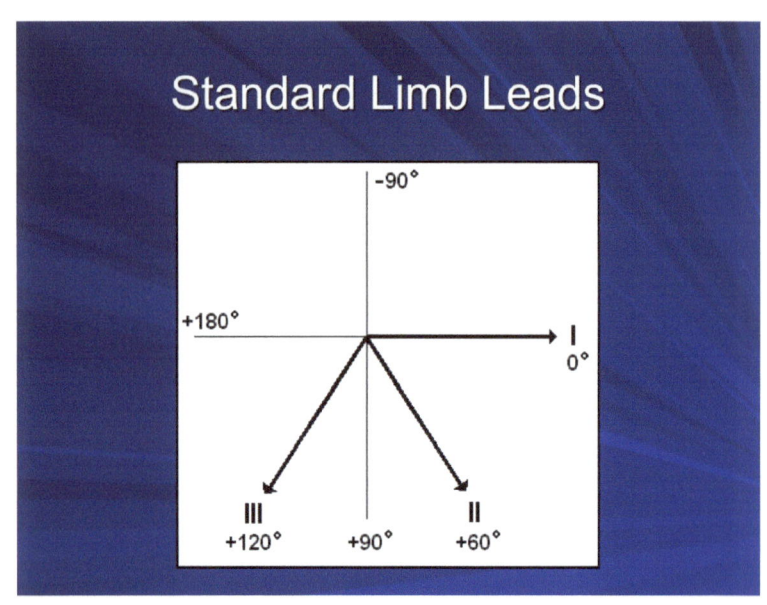

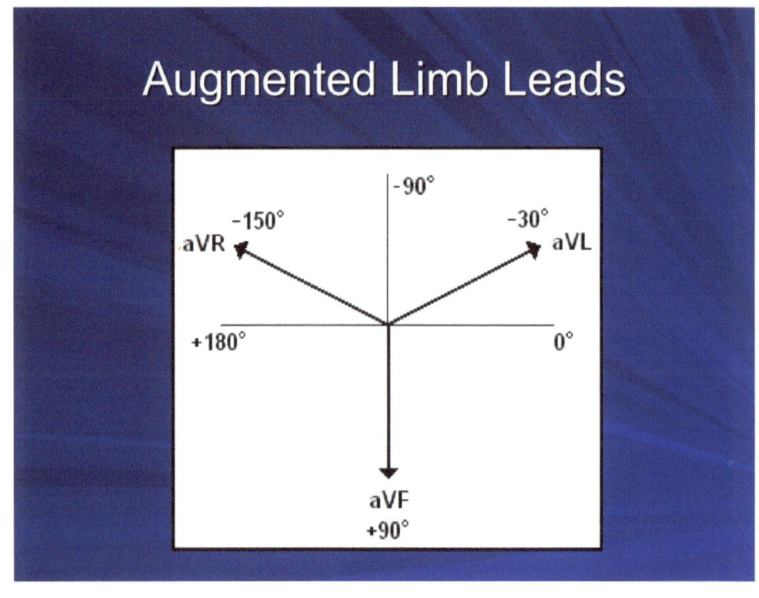

All Limb Leads

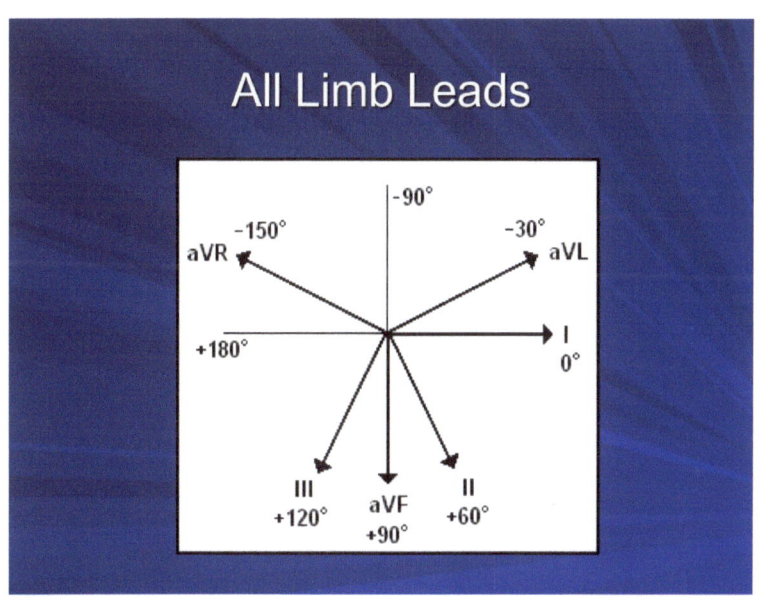

Precordial Leads

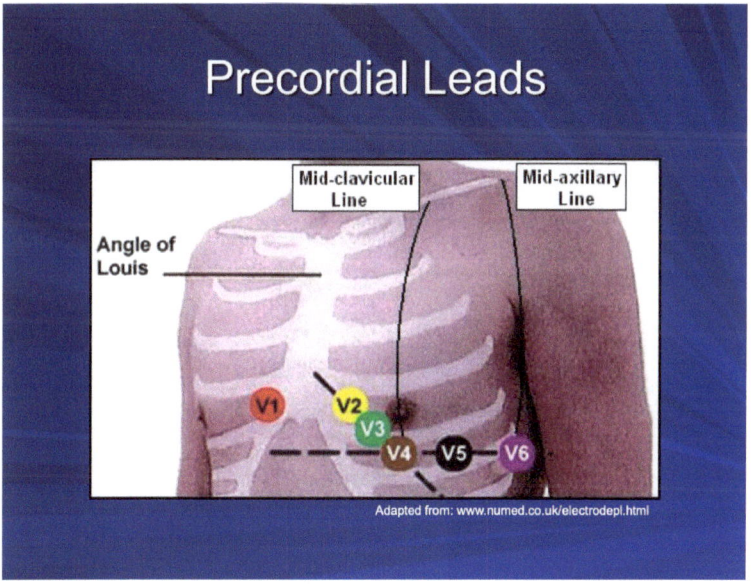

Precordial Leads

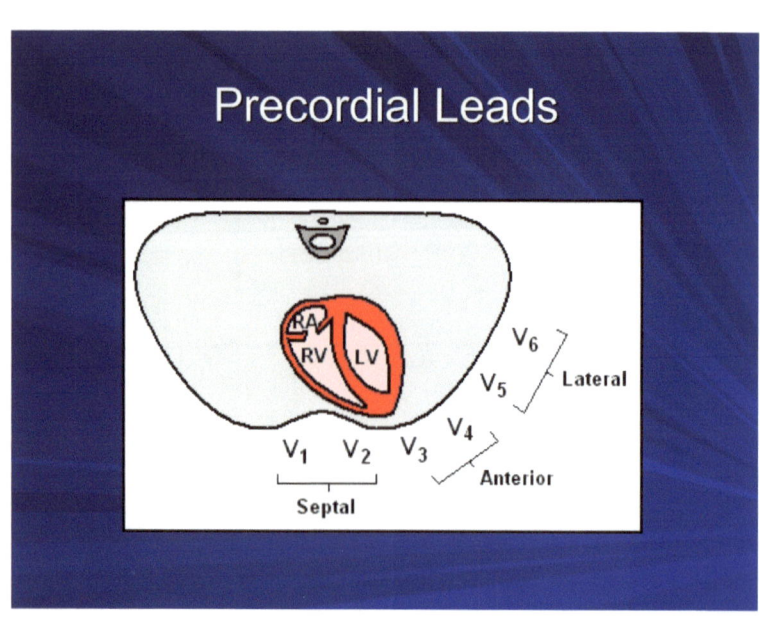

Summary of Leads

	Limb Leads	Precordial Leads
Bipolar	I, II, III (standard limb leads)	-
Unipolar	aVR, aVL, aVF (augmented limb leads)	V_1-V_6

Arrangement of Leads on the EKG

I	aVR	V_1	V_4
II	aVL	V_2	V_5
III	aVF	V_3	V_6

Arrangement of Leads on the ECG/EKG.

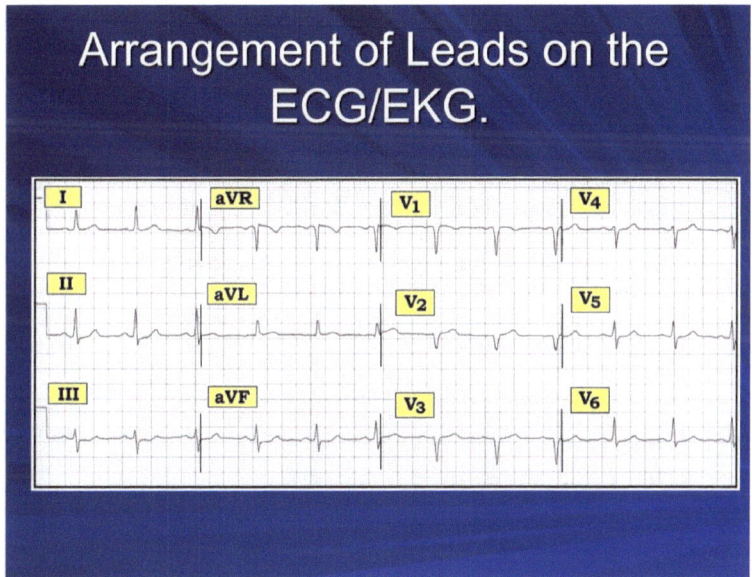

Anatomic Groups (Septum)

I Lateral	aVR None	V₁ Septal	V₄ Anterior
II Inferior	aVL Lateral	V₂ Septal	V₅ Lateral
III Inferior	aVF Inferior	V₃ Anterior	V₆ Lateral

Anatomic Groups (Anterior Wall)

I Lateral	aVR None	V₁ Septal	V₄ Anterior
II Inferior	aVL Lateral	V₂ Septal	V₅ Lateral
III Inferior	aVF Inferior	V₃ Anterior	V₆ Lateral

Anatomic Groups
(Lateral Wall)

I Lateral	aVR None	V₁ Septal	V₄ Anterior
II Inferior	aVL Lateral	V₂ Septal	V₅ Lateral
III Inferior	aVF Inferior	V₃ Anterior	V₆ Lateral

(Highlighted: I Lateral, aVL Lateral, V₅ Lateral, V₆ Lateral)

Anatomic Groups
(Inferior Wall)

I Lateral	aVR None	V₁ Septal	V₄ Anterior
II Inferior	aVL Lateral	V₂ Septal	V₅ Lateral
III Inferior	aVF Inferior	V₃ Anterior	V₆ Lateral

(Highlighted: II Inferior, III Inferior, aVF Inferior)

Anatomic Groups
(Summary)

I Lateral	aVR None	V_1 Septal	V_4 Anterior
II Inferior	aVL Lateral	V_2 Septal	V_5 Lateral
III Inferior	aVF Inferior	V_3 Anterior	V_6 Lateral

Determining the Heart Rate

- Rule of 300

- 10 Second Rule

Rule of 300

Take the number of "big boxes" between neighboring QRS complexes, and divide this into 300. The result will be approximately equal to the rate

Although fast, this method only works for regular rhythms.

What is the heart rate?

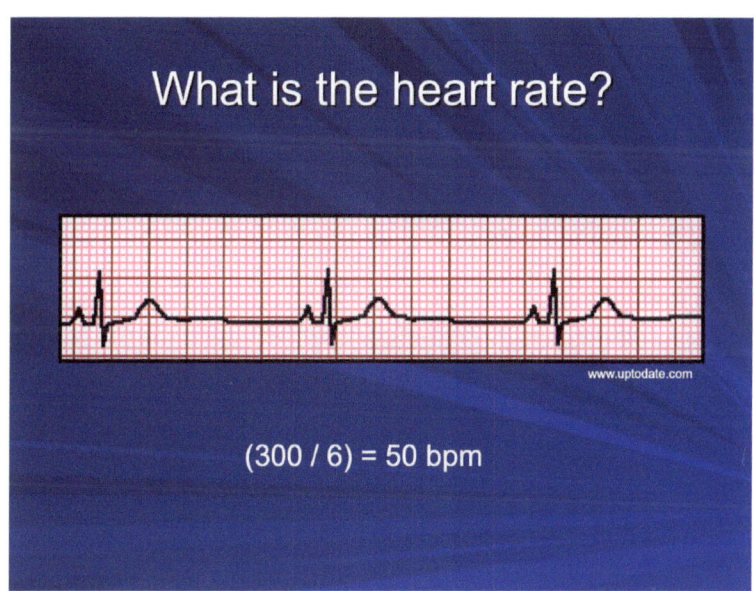

(300 / 6) = 50 bpm

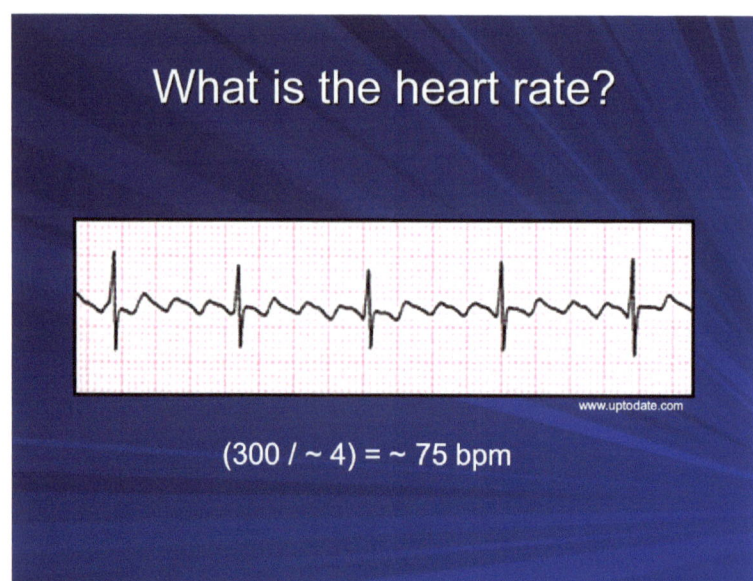

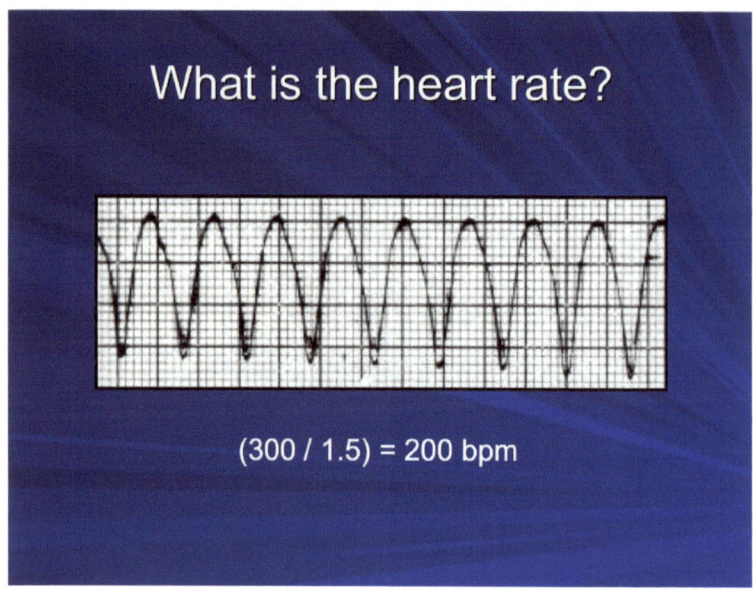

The Rule of 300

It may be easiest to memorize the following table:

# of big boxes	Rate
1	300
2	150
3	100
4	75
5	60
6	50

10 Second Rule

As most EKGs record 10 seconds of rhythm per page, one can simply count the number of beats present on the EKG and multiply by 6 to get the number of beats per 60 seconds.

This method works well for irregular rhythms.

What is the heart rate?

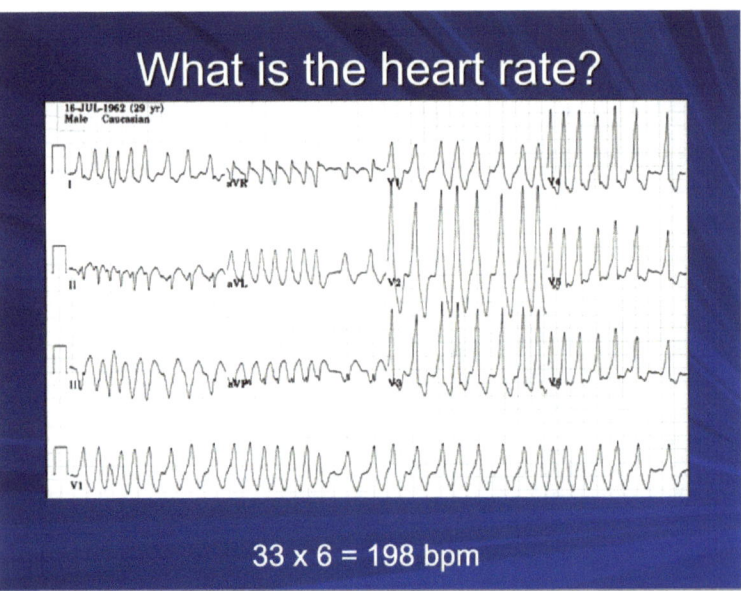

33 x 6 = 198 bpm

The QRS Axis

The QRS axis represents the net overall direction of the heart's electrical activity.

Abnormalities of axis can hint at:
- Ventricular enlargement
- Conduction blocks (i.e. hemiblocks or fascicular blocks)

The QRS Axis

By near-consensus, the normal QRS axis is defined as ranging from -30° to +90°.

-30° to -90° is referred to as a left axis deviation (LAD)

+90° to +180° is referred to as a right axis deviation (RAD)

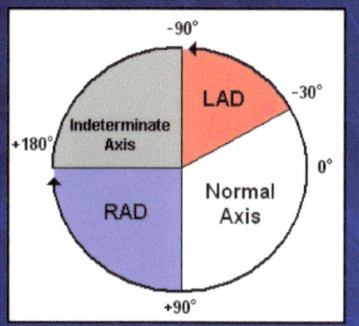

Determining the Axis

- The Quadrant Approach

- The Equiphasic Approach

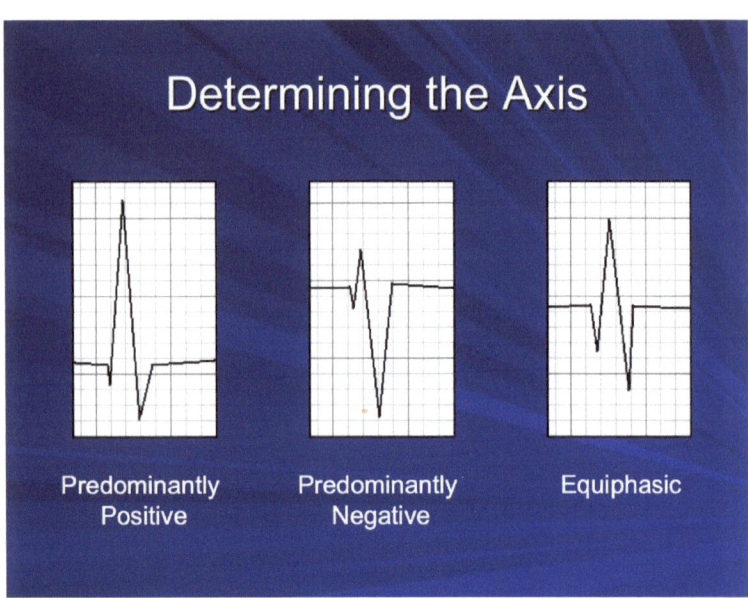

The Quadrant Approach

2. In the event that LAD is present, examine lead II to determine if this deviation is pathologic. If the QRS in II is predominantly positive, the LAD is non-pathologic (in other words, the axis is normal). If it is predominantly negative, it is pathologic.

		Lead aVF	
		Positive	Negative
Lead I	Positive	Normal Axis	LAD
	Negative	RAD	Indeterminate Axis

Quadrant Approach: Example 1

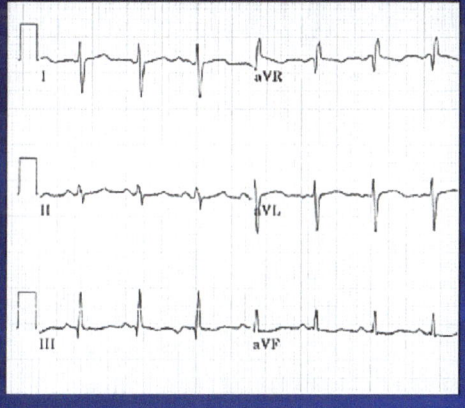

Negative in I, positive in aVF → RAD

Quadrant Approach: Example 2

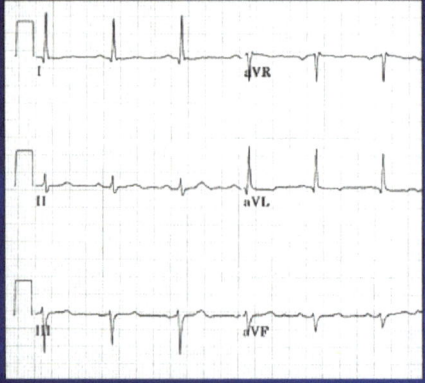

Positive in I, negative in aVF → Predominantly positive in II →
Normal Axis (non-pathologic LAD)

The Equiphasic Approach

1. Determine which lead contains the most equiphasic QRS complex. The fact that the QRS complex in this lead is equally positive and negative indicates that the net electrical vector (i.e. overall QRS axis) is perpendicular to the axis of this particular lead.

2. Examine the QRS complex in whichever lead lies 90° away from the lead identified in step 1. If the QRS complex in this second lead is predominantly positive, than the axis of this lead is approximately the same as the net QRS axis. If the QRS complex is predominantly negative, than the net QRS axis lies 180° from the axis of this lead.

Equiphasic Approach: Example 1

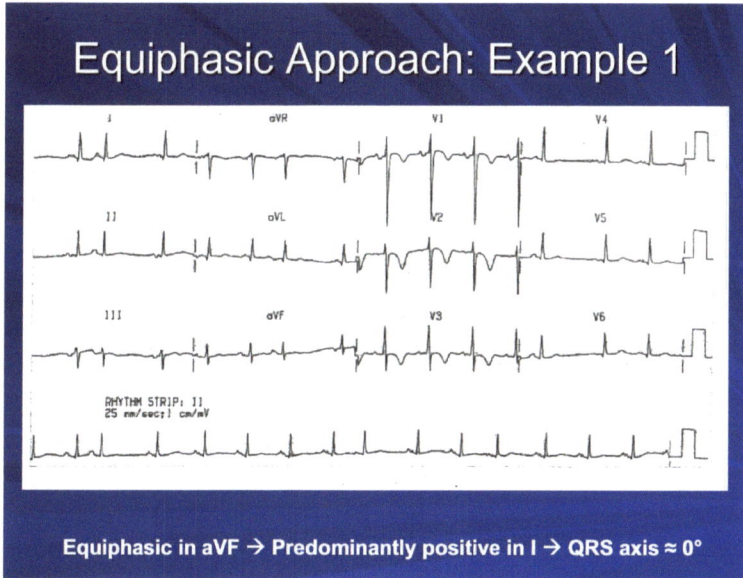

Equiphasic in aVF → Predominantly positive in I → QRS axis ≈ 0°

Equiphasic Approach: Example 2

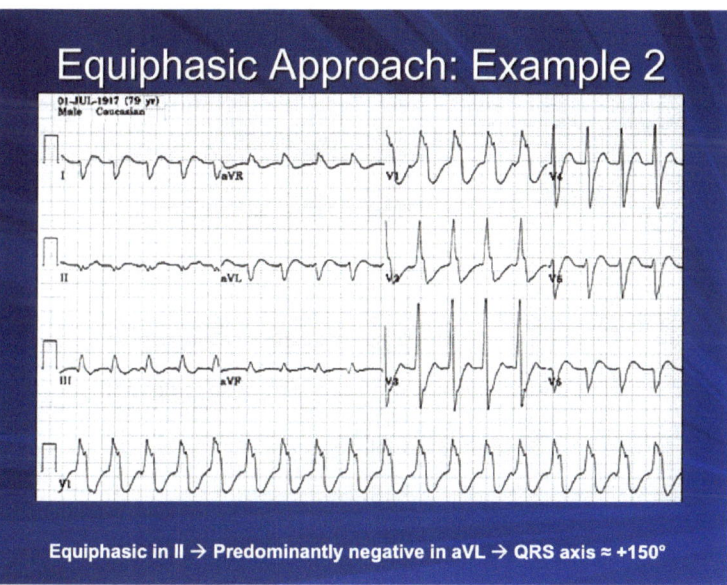

Equiphasic in II → Predominantly negative in aVL → QRS axis ≈ +150°

Basic Rhythm Problems & Their Treatment. Nodal Tissue.

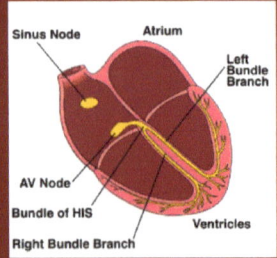

By: Dr. Richard M. Fleming
Physicist – Nuclear Cardiologist

Movement of Ions Across Cell Membranes Generate a Current, which is continued as long as the cell is alive and mitochondria are generating energy to maintain electrochemical gradient across cell membrane.

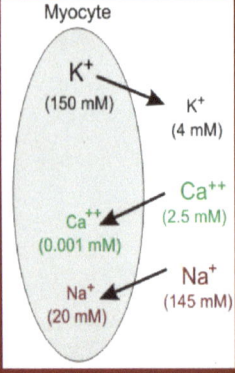
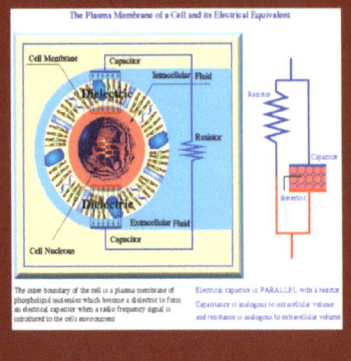

Automaticity: SA & AV node Pacemaker & Action Potential.

- The Action Potential (AP) results from:
  - Decreased outward flux of K+
  - Unchanged inward movement of Na+
  - Slow inward leak of Ca++

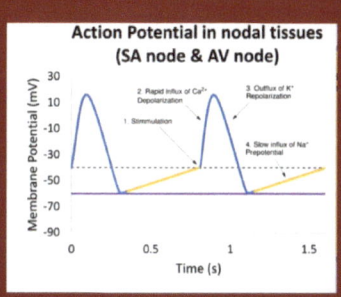

Nervous System Effect on HR.

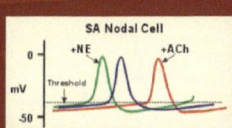

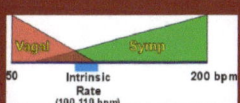

- PNS (vagal) releases Acetylcholine on SA node
  - Keeps cell Negatively charged!
    - Increases K+ (out)
    - Decreases Ca++ (in)
- SNS (inhibits vagal tone) and releases NE on SA
  - Makes cell Positively charged!
    - Decreases K+ (out)
    - Increases Ca++ (in)
    - Increases Na+ (in)

Basic Rhythm Problems & Their Treatment. His-Purkinje Tissue.

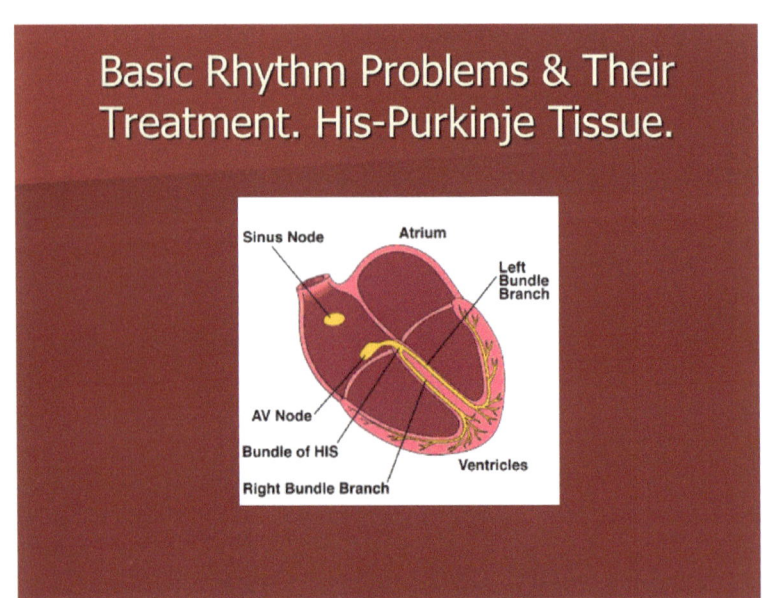

Action Potential of Bundle of His & Myocardium.

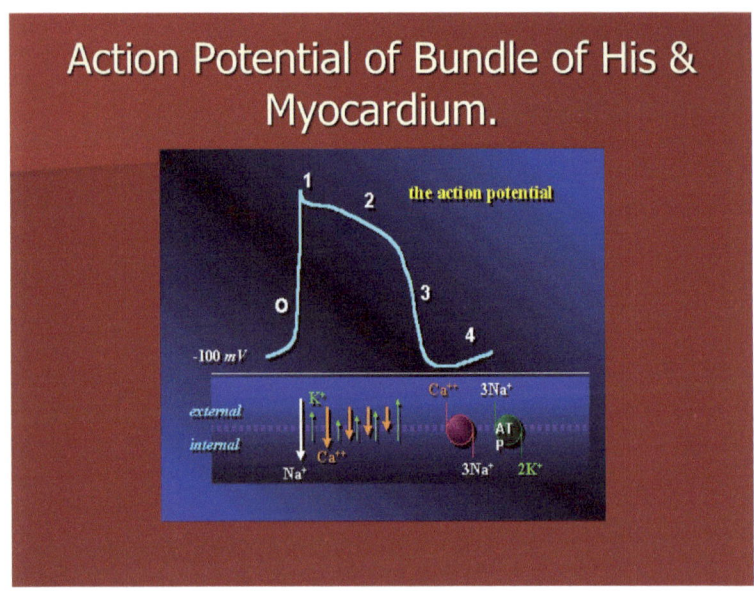

The Effect of Cardiac Drugs on Cellular Depolarization (viz. QT).

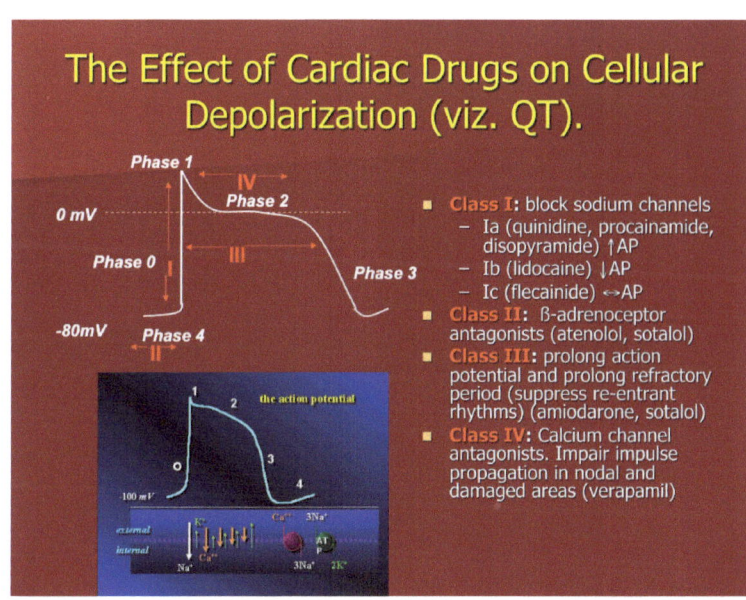

- **Class I:** block sodium channels
  - Ia (quinidine, procainamide, disopyramide) ↑AP
  - Ib (lidocaine) ↓AP
  - Ic (flecainide) ↔AP
- **Class II:** ß-adrenoceptor antagonists (atenolol, sotalol)
- **Class III:** prolong action potential and prolong refractory period (suppress re-entrant rhythms) (amiodarone, sotalol)
- **Class IV:** Calcium channel antagonists. Impair impulse propagation in nodal and damaged areas (verapamil)

Asystole

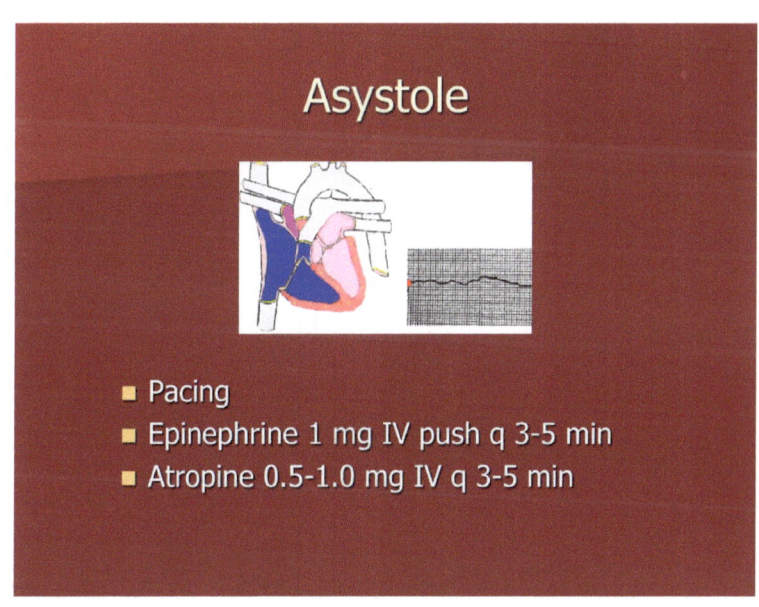

- Pacing
- Epinephrine 1 mg IV push q 3-5 min
- Atropine 0.5-1.0 mg IV q 3-5 min

What's The First Thing you Need to Do?

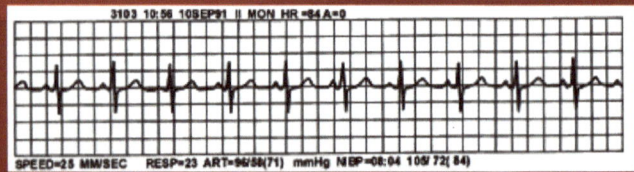

- Check the patient
  - Alert, pulse, blood pressure
- Pulseless Electrical Activity (PEA)

Pulseless Electrical Activity (PEA).

- Hypovolemia (Shock: fluid)
- Hypoxia (Oxygen)
- Acidosis (H+: bicarb or ventilation)
- Hyper or hypo-
  - Kalemia (K+: CaCl2, GIK)
- Hypothermia (warm)
- Tamponade (Pericardiocentesis)
- MI (Thrombosis: Lytics)
- Pulmonary Embolus
  - (PE Thrombus:Heparin)
- Tension Pneumothorax (Chest tube or needle)
- Tablets (Drug OD: antagonists)

Reverse the underlying causes and further treat with epinephrine and atropine.

Sinus Bradycardia

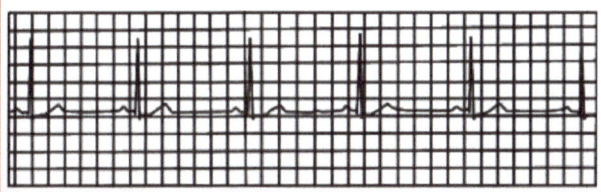

- Atropine 0.5-1.0 mg
- Epinephrine 1.0 mg
- Infusions (IV):
  - Dopamine 5-20 mic/kg/min
  - Epinephrine 2-10 mic/min
  - Isoproterenol 2-10 mic/min

Sinus Tachycardia

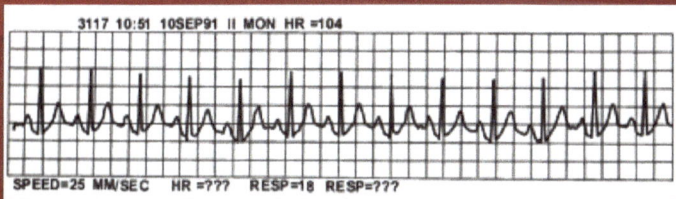

- Metoprolol 5 mg IV q 5 min x 3, then PO dose.
- Atenolol 5 mg IV over 5 min, then 10 min later repeat followed by PO dose.
- Esmolol 0.5 mg/kg load over 1 minute, then 0.05-0.3 mg/kg/min.

Basic Rhythm Problems & Their Treatment. First Degree AV Block.

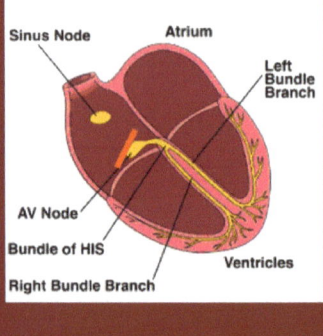

Supra-Nodal.

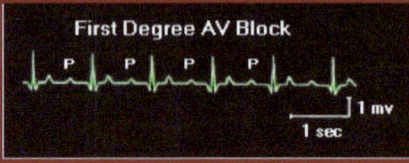

- Remove offending agents
- Atropine, pressors.

Basic Rhythm Problems & Their Treatment. Second Degree Mobitz I.

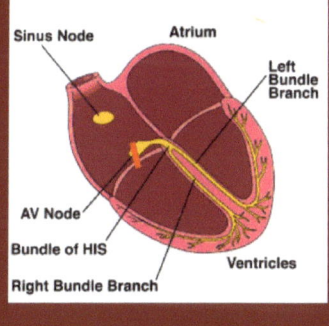

Second Degree AV Block.

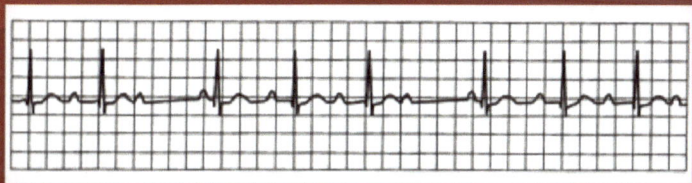

- Mobitz I (Wenckebach): AV node.
- Remove offending agents.
- Atropine, Pressors

Basic Rhythm Problems & Their Treatment. Second Degree Mobitz II.

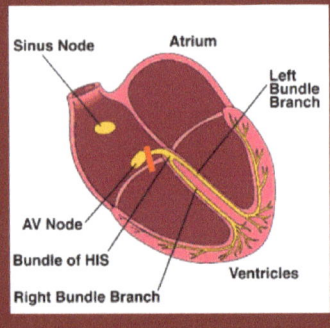

Second Degree AV Block.

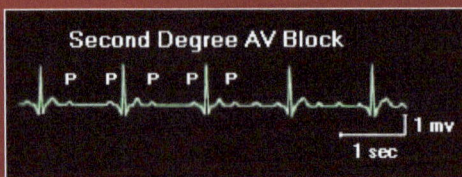

- Mobitz II (Non-Wenckebach): Infranodal
- Atropine, pressors & Pacemaker

Basic Rhythm Problems & Their Treatment. Third Degree AV Block.

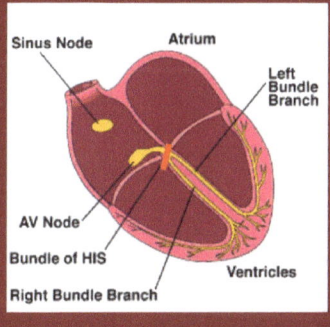

Third Degree AV Block.

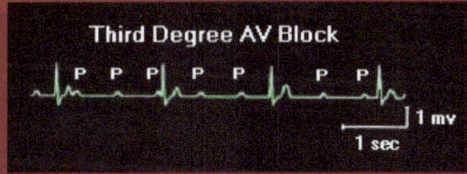

- Mobitz II (Non-Wenckebach): Infranodal
- Atropine, pressors & Pacemaker

Atrial Fibrillation.

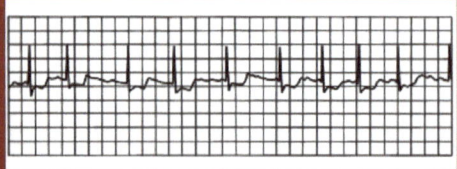

- Control Ventricular Response and Reduce Formation of Thrombus.
- Diltiazem, Propafenone, Amiodarone (300 mg IV in D5W, then 150 mg repeat, then 1 mg/min x 6 hours, then 0.5 mg/min) up to 2.2gm IV/24 hrs.

Atrial Flutter

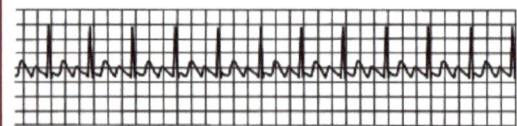

- Verapamil 2.5-5.0 mg IV over 2 minutes.
- Then 5 mg IV q 15 minutes.
- Reverse with Calcium, not fluids

Ventricular Tachycardia

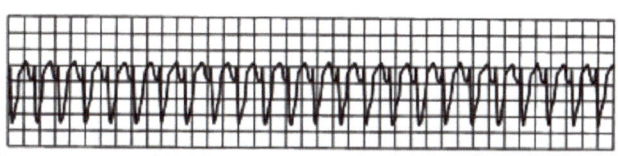

- Do not cardiovert (synchronized) until hemodynamically unstable.
- Amiodarone 150 mg IV over 10 minutes
- Lidocaine 0.5-0.75 mg/kg IV push
- Sotalol 1-1.5 mg/kg @ 10 mg/min
- Procainamide 17 mg/kg @ 20 mg/min (then 1-4 mg/min)

R on T Phenomena -> VT

Characteristic ECG features

Pause / Short-Long-Short sequence

Non-pause

T-wave alternans

Common mechanism of arrhythmia initiation

"R-from-T"

Torsade de Pointe

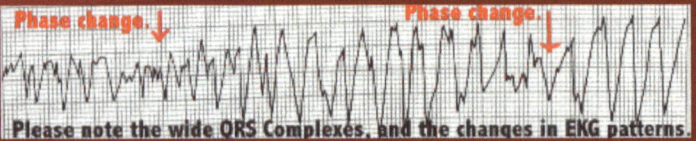

- Remove offending agents
  - IA: Quinidine, Procainamide, Disopyramide
- Magnesium, DPH
- Overdrive pacing with pacemaker or isoprel.

Ventricular Fibrillation

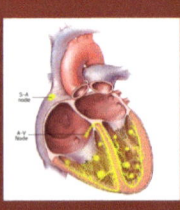 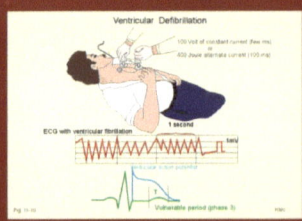

- Cardiovert (non-synchronized)
- Amiodarone 150 mg IV over 10 minutes
- Lidocaine 0.5-0.75 mg/kg IV push
- Sotalol 1-1.5 mg/kg @ 10 mg/min
- Procainamide 17 mg/kg @ 20 mg/min (then 1-4 mg/min)

Dysrhythmias and EKGs

(Arrhythmia = Asystole or the absence of a rhythm.)

By: Dr. Richard M. Fleming
Physicist – Nuclear Cardiologist

Outline

1. Normal Sinus Rhythm
2. Altered Automaticity
3. Reentry
4. Conduction Block
5. Helpful hints for diagnosing arrhythmias

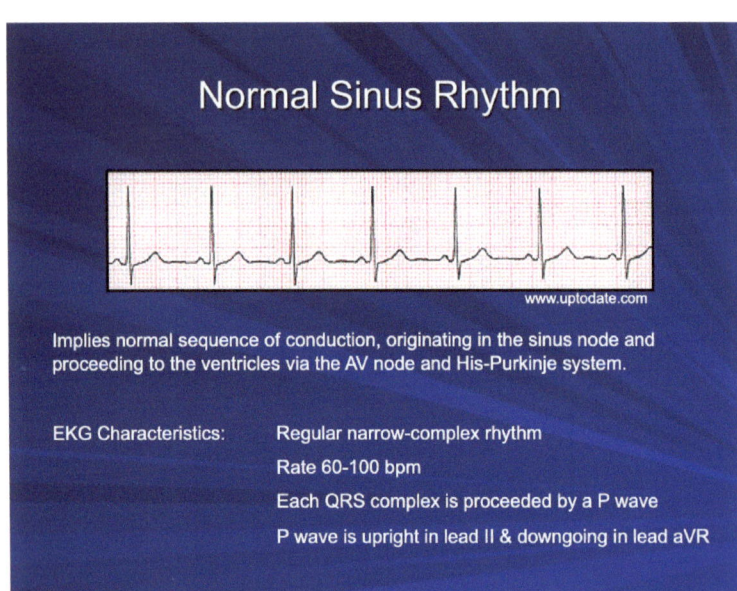

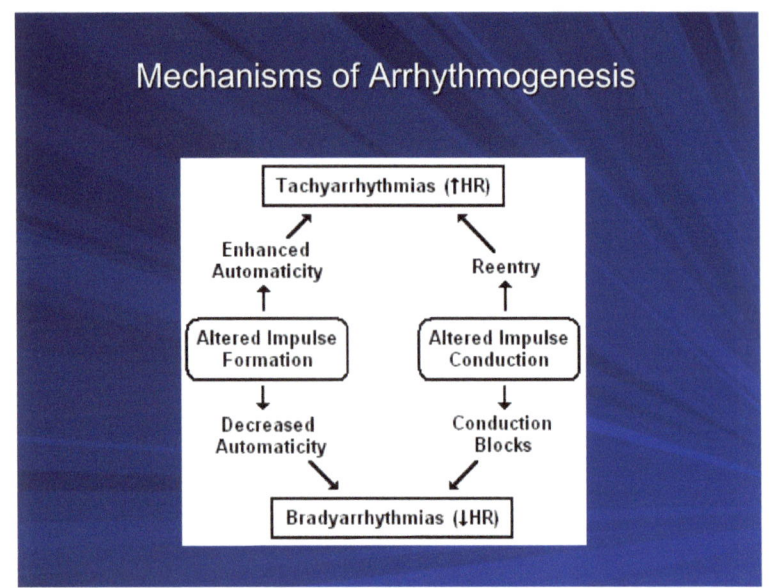

Recognizing altered automaticity on EKG

Gradual onset and termination of the arrhythmia.

The P wave of the first beat of the arrhythmia is typically the same as the remaining beats of the arrhythmia (if a P wave is present at all).

Decreased Automaticity

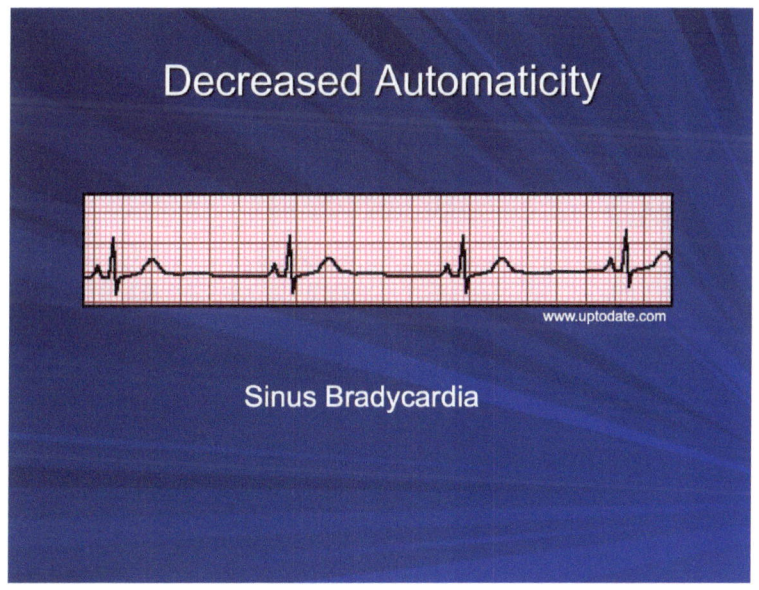

Sinus Bradycardia

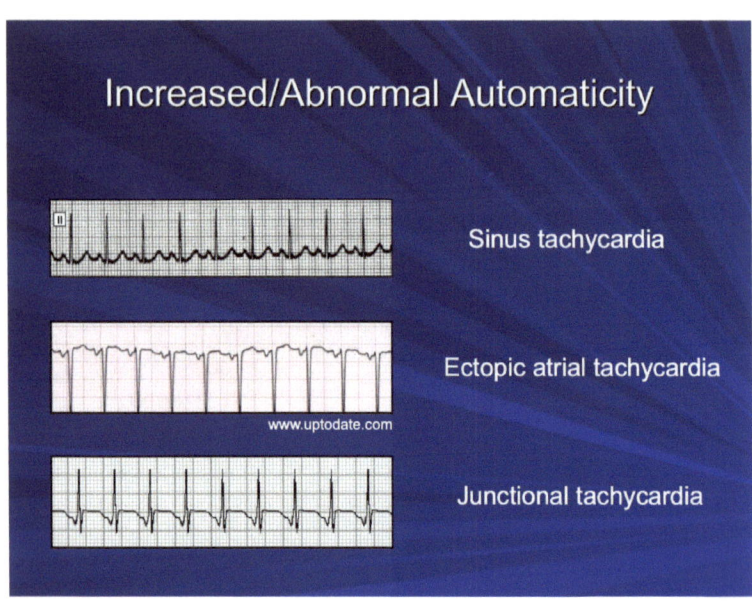

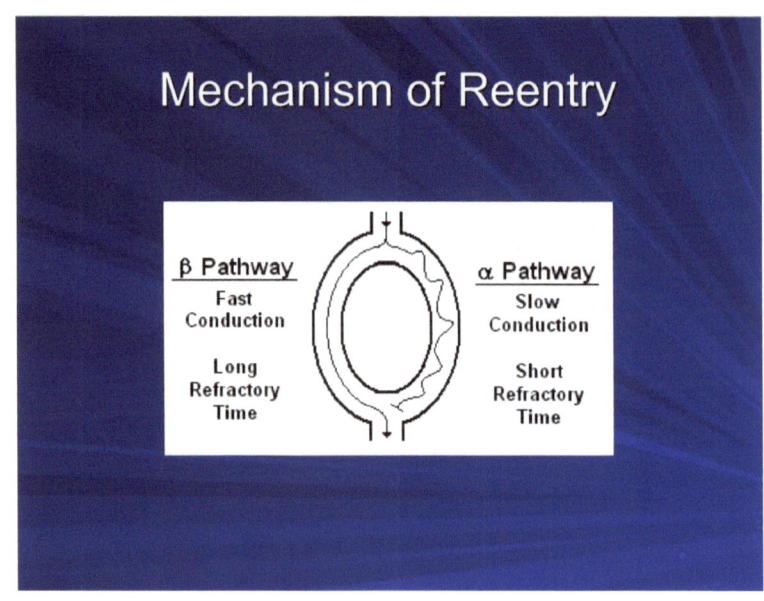

Mechanism of Reentry

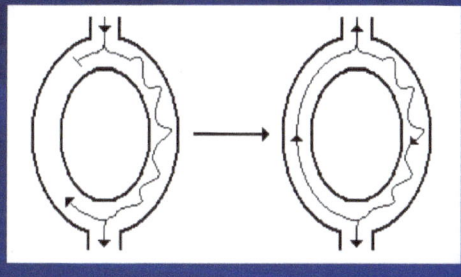

Reentrant Rhythms

- AV nodal reentrant tachycardia (AVNRT)
- AV reentrant tachycardia (AVRT)
  - Orthodromic
  - Antidromic
- Atrial flutter
- Atrial fibrillation
- Ventricular tachycardia

Recognizing reentry on EKG

Abrupt onset and termination of the arrhythmia.

The P wave of the first beat of the arrhythmia is different as the remaining beats of the arrhythmia (if a P wave is present at all).

Example of AVNRT

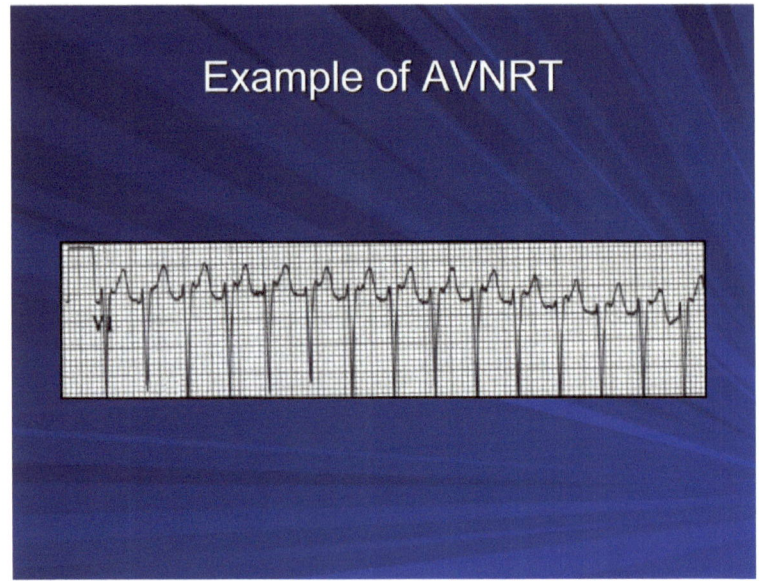

Mechanism of AVNRT

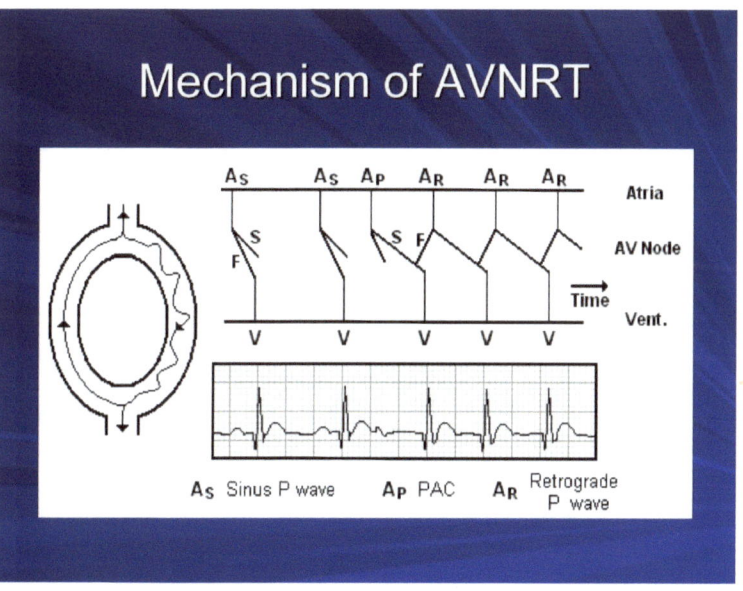

Atrial Flutter

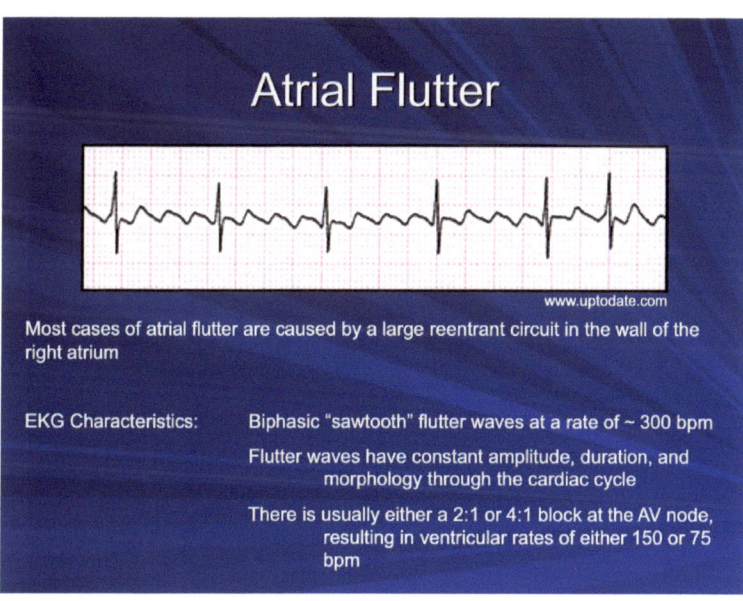

Most cases of atrial flutter are caused by a large reentrant circuit in the wall of the right atrium

EKG Characteristics: Biphasic "sawtooth" flutter waves at a rate of ~ 300 bpm

Flutter waves have constant amplitude, duration, and morphology through the cardiac cycle

There is usually either a 2:1 or 4:1 block at the AV node, resulting in ventricular rates of either 150 or 75 bpm

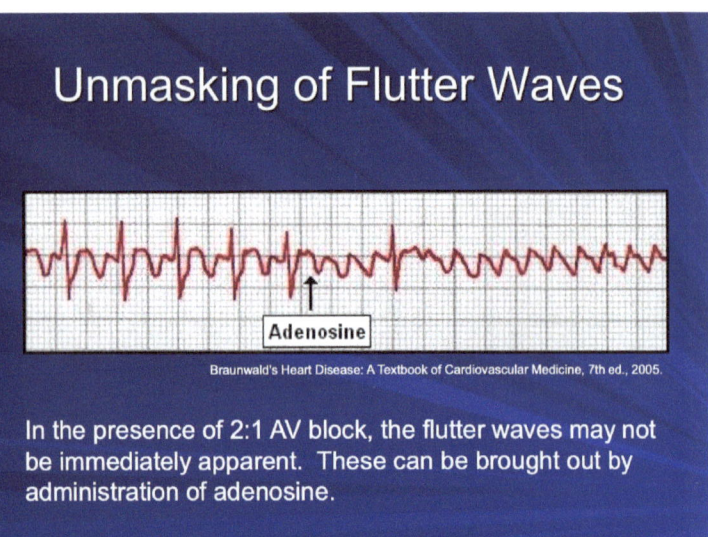

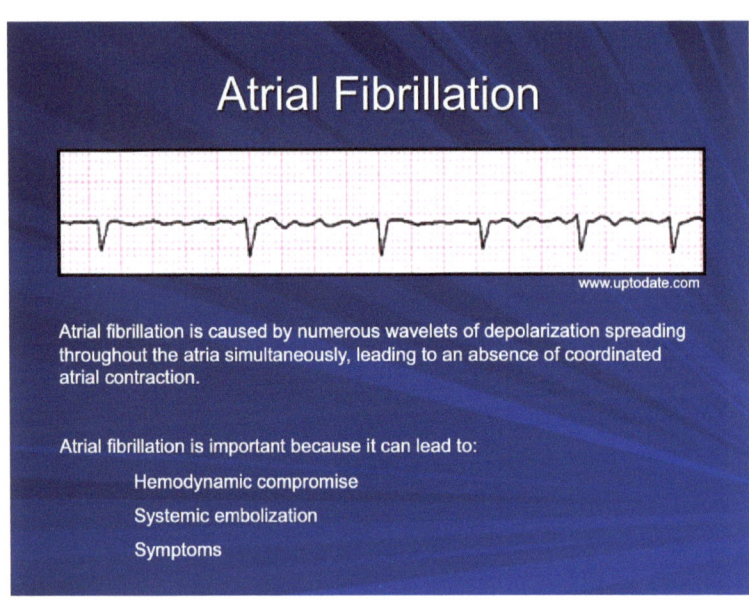

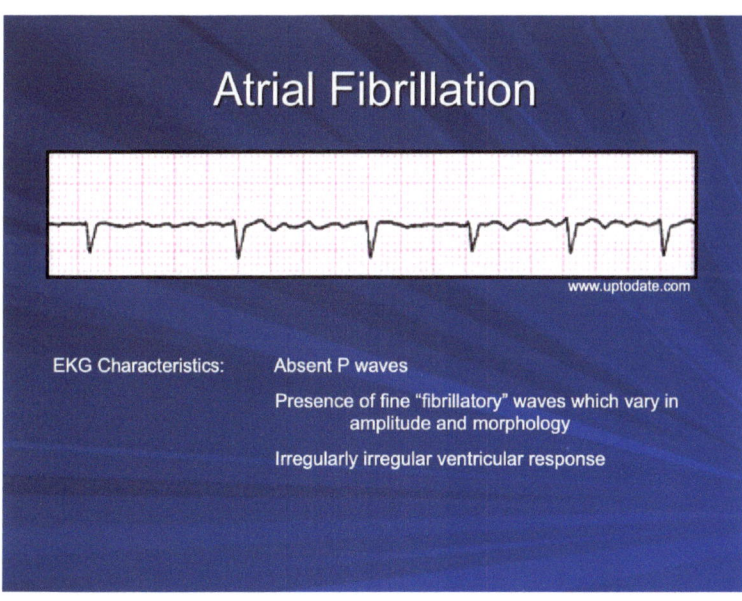
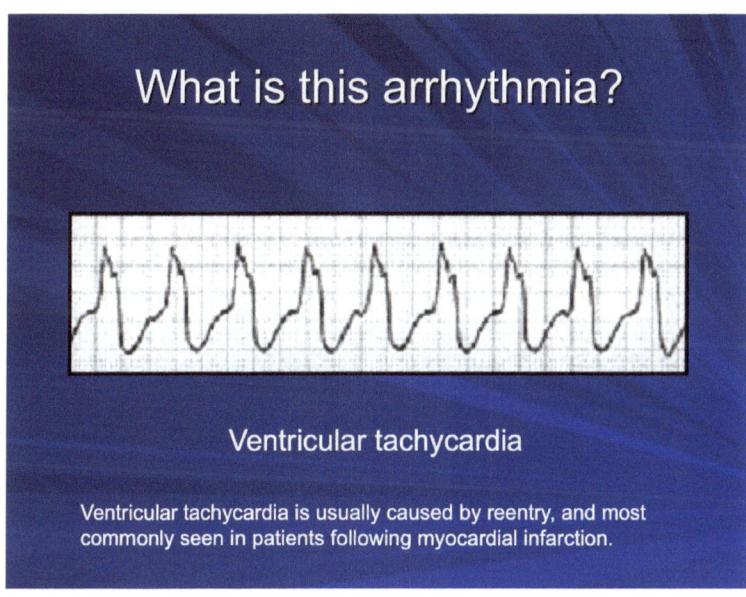

Rhythms Produced by Conduction Block

- AV Block (relatively common)
  - 1st degree AV block
  - Type 1 2nd degree AV block
  - Type 2 2nd degree AV block
  - 3rd degree AV block

- SA Block (relatively rare)

1st Degree AV Block

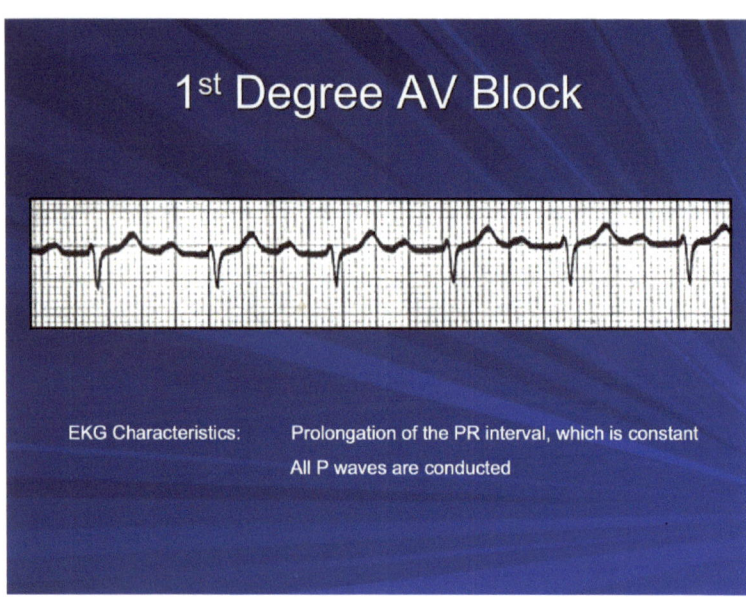

EKG Characteristics: Prolongation of the PR interval, which is constant
All P waves are conducted

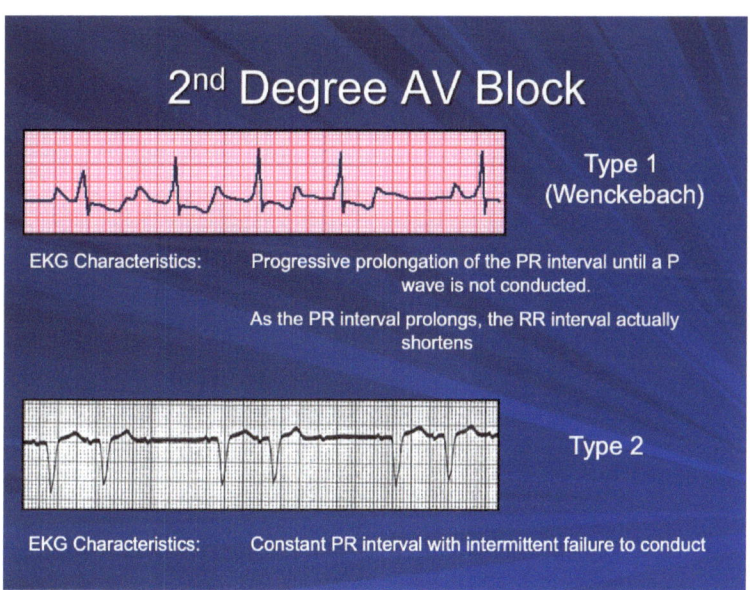

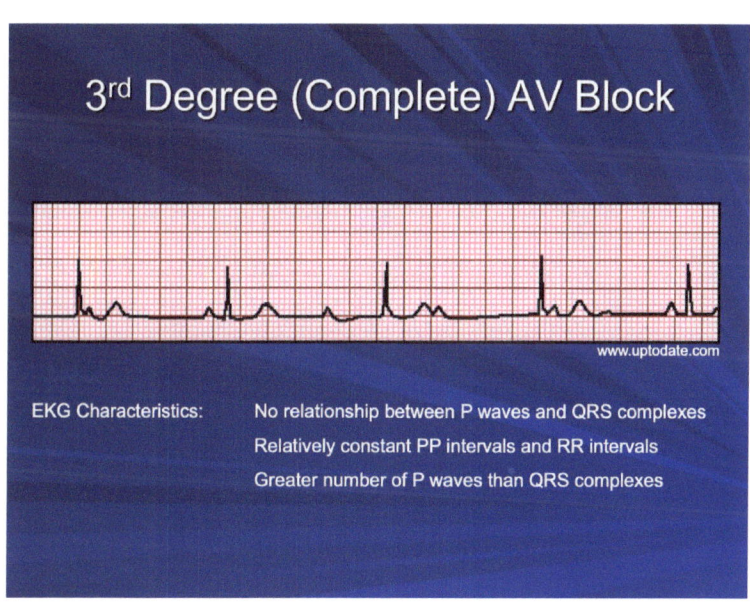

Questions to answer in order to identify an unknown arrhythmia:

1. Is the rate slow (<60 bpm) or fast (>100 bpm)?
   Slow → Suggests sinus bradycardia, sinus arrest, or conduction block
   Fast → Suggests increased/abnormal automaticity or reentry

2. Is the rhythm irregular?
   Irregular → Suggests atrial fibrillation, 2nd degree AV block, multifocal atrial tachycardia, or atrial flutter with variable AV block

3. Is the QRS complex narrow or wide?
   Narrow → Rhythm must originate from the AV node or above
   Wide → Rhythm may originate from anywhere

Questions to answer in order to identify an unknown arrhythmia:

4. Are there P waves?
   Absent P waves → Suggests atrial fibrillation, ventricular tachycardia, or rhythms originating from the AV node

5. What is the relationship between the P waves and QRS complexes?
   More P waves than QRS complexes → Suggests 2nd or 3rd degree AV block
   More QRS complexes than P waves → Suggests an accelerated junctional or ventricular rhythm

6. Is the onset/termination of the rhythm abrupt or gradual?
   Abrupt → Suggests reentrant rhythm
   Gradual → Suggests altered automaticity

The importance of learning how to read rhythm disturbances if far more than just being able to answer questions correctly on a test, or even being able to demonstrate to others that you can read electrocardiograms.

Electrocardiograms are obtained to look for specific problems with the heart, and with that knowledge to know what treatments to prescribe to address each patient's specific cardiac problem. This includes which drugs or treatments to provide to control the patient's heart rate and when combined with proper control and treatment of their blood pressure, improvement in their stroke volume, and their overall cardiac output.

www.ingramcontent.com/pod-product-compliance
Lightning Source LLC
Chambersburg PA
CBHW040246220526
45473CB00001B/387